Livin

CW01510282

Gluten

Intolerance

How to Enjoy Living
Gluten Free!

Jennifer Williams

Disclaimer

The content of this book is for informational purposes only. It's not meant to be a substitute for proper medical diagnosis, treatment or advice, and you should not assume that it is. If you or someone you know suspects they have gluten intolerance, it's essential to consult with a healthcare professional for proper diagnosis and management. Always consult with your healthcare provider before taking any medications, natural remedies, supplements, or making any major changes to your diet.

CONTENTS

1. INTRODUCTION

When you first learned that you had gluten intolerance you most likely felt desperate, scared, and even angry because you thought your world had come to an end. But it certainly has not.

Like many people in your position, you might have felt a real sense of relief that, at long last, you now knew why you'd been feeling so bad for so long, and that it hadn't been "all in your head" as you'd probably been told on more than one occasion.

Think about that for a moment; you now know exactly why you've been feeling so ill and "down" for so long.

Isn't that a positive thing? Of course it is, because now that you've been diagnosed you can work towards a brand new you: happy, healthy, gregarious, and full of energy!

So, in this concise book, in clear and simple language, you'll discover:

- the basics about your condition and why you need to eliminate gluten entirely.

- how to recognize your food friends and food enemies.

- how to stay gluten-free indoors and out.

- the 6 simple steps to going gluten-free.

- how to handle food cravings.

- how to deal with accidental gluten ingestion.

- weekly gluten-free meal plans.

- affirmations to give yourself a mental boost.

- useful resources.

2. DO WE NEED GLUTEN?

Gluten is a protein found in wheat, barley and rye. It's what makes the dough so elastic after kneading and helps baked goods keep their shape by trapping and preventing gas from escaping during the baking process.

It's also used as an additive in some foods that would otherwise be low in protein and as a stabilizing agent in certain other foods.

So since gluten is a protein we need it, right? No. Although it's a protein, the amount of protein we get from wheat, barley and rye is a good deal lower than we can get from a whole variety of other foods.

For example, bread has between 6.70 to 11.40 grams of protein per 100 grams, while cooked meat has between 16.90 and 40.60. Parmesan cheese has 34.99 to 40.79 and peanuts 23.68 to 28.04. So we don't need gluten as there are many other, richer, sources of protein.

However, whole grains provide us with valuable nutrients such as vitamins, minerals, and fiber. So their overall health benefit shouldn't be ignored, although it has to be recognized that these nutrients can also be found in a wide range of gluten-free foods.

On balance then, although we can live without gluten, whole grains are beneficial to most of us, albeit there's an increasing number of people who choose to cut gluten, and therefore grains, from their diet.

Unfortunately, for those who suffer from gluten intolerance, there isn't a free choice, as gluten can make them sick. If you have gluten intolerance then you know this very well.

The important thing is that, whatever your reason is for going gluten-free, you need to ensure that you replace those lost nutrients in a healthy, well-balanced diet.

3. INTOLERANCE, SENSITIVITY AND ALLERGY

A lot of the time even some professionals use the words "intolerance," "sensitivity" and "allergy" interchangeably. But this is quite wrong as the underlying mechanisms are different.

While intolerance and sensitivity are basically the same thing, an allergy causes a different reaction in the body.

Allergy

More and more people are becoming allergic to things like food, skin products, dust, pollen, animal hair, and a myriad of other items they are exposed to in their everyday lives.

An allergic reaction to food, for example, occurs when the body "believes" a specific part of the food (usually a protein) is harmful and so triggers an immune response to fight the food "allergen."

This produces antibodies which, in turn, produce certain chemicals such as histamine that cause adverse reactions in the body, affecting areas like the skin, stomach, breathing and heart.

A first-time exposure to an allergen may only result in a relatively mild reaction, but repeated exposures usually result in increasingly severe reactions.

An allergic reaction can be so severe that it can even lead to life-threatening anaphylactic shock.

Allergic reactions usually come on rather quickly; seconds or minutes after exposure. However, in some cases, it can take several hours, especially where the allergen has been digested.

Intolerance/Sensitivity

When someone has intolerance or sensitivity to a certain food it means they suffer an adverse reaction to ingesting it.

However, the intolerance isn't due to the immune system response that causes an allergy. Rather, it occurs because the patient's digestive system can't tolerate the food in question. Several non-allergenic mechanisms can cause this, which is why its medical name is "non-allergic food hypersensitivity."

Food intolerance is much more prevalent than food allergy. The signs of intolerance normally come on more slowly than an allergic reaction, perhaps 12 to 24 hours after exposure, although they may show up almost immediately in some specific cases.

4. WHAT IS GLUTEN INTOLERANCE

Gluten intolerance is often used to describe the condition where a person has "sensitivity" to gluten but does not have celiac disease – mostly spelt "coeliac disease" outside North America.

Unfortunately, gluten intolerance is also very often used as a catch-all to describe various gluten-related conditions, including celiac disease and gluten sensitivity, or more correctly, non-celiac gluten sensitivity.

To make matters even worse, sometimes wheat allergy is included under the gluten intolerance banner too. This is misleading since many proteins in wheat can cause an allergy. And, as you have already seen, allergy is not the same as intolerance.

So using gluten intolerance to encapsulate all gluten-related issues may not be helpful as it's perhaps too general a term.

The following two chapters will explain the important differences between celiac disease and non-celiac gluten sensitivity which often come together under the banner of "gluten intolerance."

5. CELIAC DISEASE

Celiac disease – also known as "gluten-sensitive enteropathy" and "celiac sprue" – is a genetic autoimmune disorder that affects 1 in 100 people worldwide. The genetic component means that someone with celiac disease in their immediate family has a 1 in 10 risk of developing the disease.

It affects males and females of all ages and races who have specific hereditary genes that predispose them to the disease. According to Dr. Sheila Crowe, a professor in the Department of Medicine, University of Virginia, it's virtually impossible to get celiac disease without these particular genes.

It can be triggered, or become active for the first time, in someone who has had surgery, is pregnant, has given birth, has had a viral infection, or has severe emotional stress.

It has many of the features of a food allergy but isn't caused by an immune system response; it's caused by an "autoimmune" response.

Whereas an immune response attacks the perceived allergen, an autoimmune response is where the immune system malfunctions and mistakenly attacks the body's tissue which, in the case of a celiac, is the lining of their small intestine.

The lining is covered in small finger-like protrusions called "villi" which increase the effective surface area of the small intestine to help optimize the passage of nutrients into the bloodstream at the correct absorption rate.

In a celiac, the villi are damaged and flattened by the autoimmune response – "villous atrophy" – thus reducing the body's ability to absorb correctly the nutrients, vitamins and minerals from ingested food. This leads to malnutrition and a host of other serious health conditions.

Celiac Disease and Related Health Conditions

If not addressed, celiac disease can lead to other serious health issues such as:

- malnutrition

- miscarriage

- infertility

- osteoporosis

- anemia

- low-bone density

- iron deficiency

- thyroid problems

- lupus

- type 1 diabetes

- rheumatoid arthritis

- increased risk of non-Hodgkin lymphoma

The lining can even become permeable or "leaky," allowing food particles and toxins to enter the bloodstream with the risk of further complications such as:

- eczema

- hives

- chronic fatigue

- aching/swelling joints

- lactose intolerance

- mental fuzziness

- mood swings

- irritable bowel syndrome (IBS)

- Crohn's disease

- colitis

Symptoms of Celiac Disease

Although the classic symptoms are weight loss and diarrhea, according to the Mayo Clinic only about a third of patients with celiac disease have diarrhea, and about half suffer weight loss. They also find that 20% of celiacs have constipation and 10% are obese.

The symptoms can vary enormously across celiac sufferers. According to the University of Chicago, Celiac Disease Center, there are some 300 symptoms associated with the disease.

However, the symptoms are not specific to celiac disease or the digestive system. And that, along with the variance across patients, makes diagnosis difficult. To make it even more difficult, many patients do not exhibit any symptoms at all!

It should be noted that those who have the disease, but show no symptoms, are still at risk of the same long-term complications as those who do display symptoms.

Symptoms of Celiac Disease in Adults

Excluding the classic symptoms of diarrhea and weight loss discussed above, the Celiac Disease Foundation lists some of the most common symptoms in adults as:

- anemia (iron deficiency)

- arthritis

- anxiety

- depression

- sores inside the mouth

- dermatitis herpetiformis (itchy skin rash)

- osteoporosis

- painful joints

- fatigue

- migraines

- infertility

- miscarriages

- missed menstrual periods

As well as the above, the Mayo Clinic also lists:

- dental enamel damage

- hyposplenism (reduced spleen function)

- acid reflux/heartburn

Celiac Disease Symptoms in Children

Children generally display more digestive symptoms than adults with celiac disease. Typical symptoms of celiac disease in children are:

- weight loss

- bloating

- abdominal pain

- frequent diarrhea

- pale, smelly stools

- constipation

- vomiting

- headaches

- behavioral problems

- frequent irritability

- fatigue

- delayed puberty and growth

- failure to thrive

- short of stature

- ADHD (Attention Deficit Hyperactivity Disorder)

- learning disability

- poor muscle coordination

6. NON-CELIAC GLUTEN SENSITIVITY

No one knows how many people there are in the world with non-celiac gluten sensitivity but there are estimates that put the figure as high as 6 out of 100 and climbing. That's 6 times the number with celiac disease.

Somebody with non-celiac gluten sensitivity – often referred to as "gluten intolerance" or "gluten sensitivity" – doesn't have the celiac genes and their immune system doesn't attack their body's tissue.

So there are none of the antibodies associated with celiac disease and their digestive system won't show any physical damage, but they can suffer similar symptoms. In other words, eating gluten can make them ill too.

Non-celiac gluten sensitivity isn't nearly as well defined as celiac disease and doesn't have a recognized diagnosis, so much less is known about the condition. Because of this, it has often been labeled as something akin to a "fad" by many in the medical profession, and not a condition at all.

However, as we learn more about it, there seems to be a gradual change in that perception, especially given its increasing prevalence. For example, a Mayo

Clinic study found a significant increase not only in celiac disease but also in non-celiac gluten sensitivity over the past 50 years.

Some put the increase in gluten sensitivity down to the type of wheat we eat today compared with what we ate 50 years ago...

The hybridized wheat of today is more processed and has additives to make it hardier, more drought resistant, to bake more easily, to keep its shape better, and so on. They believe that the human body hasn't been able to adapt to these changes. However, others dispute this.

Some experts believe that the mechanism that triggers non-celiac gluten sensitivity is an "innate immune response." This is the body's very basic, first-line response to foreign invaders.

It isn't antigen-specific and not capable of "memorizing" antigens and learning how to deal with them. And it doesn't attack the body's own tissue. So it isn't the same as an allergic immune response or the celiac autoimmune response.

Compared to celiac disease there is so much that is unknown about non-celiac gluten sensitivity. A lot more research is needed to fully understand the underlying mechanisms and risk factors.

Non-Celiac Gluten Sensitivity Symptoms

Non-celiac gluten sensitivity has many of the symptoms of celiac disease (see earlier list), with the ones outside the intestinal tract being particularly prevalent, compared to celiac disease, according to Dr. Alessio Fasano MD, at the time Head of the University of Maryland Center for Celiac Research.

According to Dr. Fasano, there are headaches, migraines and brain fog in one-third of patients diagnosed with non-celiac gluten sensitivity which, he says, is far more than in celiac patients.

Dr. Fasano also revealed that many patients diagnosed with gluten sensitivity exhibited several different eczema-like skin conditions, not just the dermatitis herpetiformis usually associated with celiac disease. His gluten-sensitive patients also reported feelings of anxiety and depression.

However, intestinal problems are still very common. Dr. Fasano says that patients report symptoms similar to Irritable Bowel Syndrome (IBS), such as diarrhea, stomach ache and bloating.

Because there are so many symptoms overlap between celiac disease and non-celiac gluten sensitivity, and other conditions such as IBS, it's impossible to diagnose either based on symptoms alone.

7. DIAGNOSIS

Testing for Celiac Disease

Celiac disease is a "multi-system" disorder which means that the symptoms can affect any part of the body. Not only that, symptoms can vary a lot between patients. This makes it impossible to make a diagnosis based only on the symptoms.

But given the presence of symptoms and where your doctor suspects you may have celiac disease – after having ruled out other potential conditions including wheat allergy – they will probably arrange for one or more blood tests to look for the antibodies associated with the disease.

However, the problem with these blood tests is that they can sometimes show up negative for the antibodies even where the disease is present.

Because of this, your doctor will most probably also arrange for an endoscopy and a biopsy of the inner lining of the intestine to ascertain if there is any damage present. And that would be the clincher, not necessarily the blood tests by themselves.

Testing for Non-Celiac Gluten Sensitivity

Unfortunately, there isn't a clinical test for gluten sensitivity as yet. So, where someone is showing a reaction to gluten, and celiac disease and wheat allergy have been ruled out, non-celiac gluten sensitivity may be considered a possibility.

After ruling out celiac disease and wheat allergy, one way that non-celiac gluten sensitivity may be indicated is through an exclusion diet...

In this process, gluten is completely removed from the diet and the patient's health is tracked to see if the symptoms improve over time, then gluten is gradually added back into their diet to see if the symptoms reappear. If this is the case then, taken together with the exclusion of celiac disease and wheat allergy earlier, the doctor may diagnose non-celiac gluten sensitivity.

Note: The above test can only work if the patient is still taking gluten in their diet at the start of the test since it depends on first removing gluten, tracking the results, and then adding gluten back into their diet to see if the symptoms return.

So, if you suspect that you might have a gluten problem, don't go onto a gluten-free diet before seeing your doctor. Continue eating as you are, consult with your doctor, and follow their instructions.

Gluten Intolerance is Underdiagnosed

Research by the University of Nottingham, England, and published in the American Journal of Gastroenterology, highlights that, although the rate at which patients are diagnosed with celiac disease has increased four-fold over the past 20 years, the percentage still going undiagnosed is 76%, representing some 500,000 people in the UK.

This is a truly shocking figure, but it's a similar story in North America; according to the National Foundation for Celiac Awareness, around 83% of sufferers don't know they have the disease.

According to Daniel Leffler, MD, MS, The Celiac Center, Beth Israel Deaconess Medical Center, the average time it takes for a person to be correctly diagnosed is 6-10 years. The Canadian Celiac Health Survey reported a mean delay of 11.7 years!

One of the reasons for this underdiagnosis may be the misdiagnosis of celiac disease for other health conditions that the symptoms share, for example, IBS.

In terms of non-celiac gluten sensitivity, the under-reporting must be way higher simply because the condition is not nearly as well defined as celiac disease and there is still skepticism within some in the medical profession that it actually exists at all.

8. IS THERE A CURE?

Unfortunately, there isn't a cure. Several ongoing studies are looking at things like enzyme therapies and immunotherapies but none have established a cure as yet.

The only way that someone who reacts negatively to gluten can get healthy again is to remove gluten from their life.

When gluten is completely removed, and the patient remains gluten-free, their body can begin to repair itself and their symptoms and other related conditions usually disappear over time.

However, there are some with celiac disease whose internal damage is so severe that going gluten-free won't repair the damage completely. They need medical help, such as nutritional supplements given intravenously, in addition to their gluten-free diet.

So a gluten-free diet isn't a lifestyle choice for people with gluten intolerance, it's a quality of life choice.

9. STEPS TO GOING GLUTEN-FREE

First off, don't worry, going gluten-free need not be as difficult as you might imagine, as long as you adopt the right mindset and take the right steps.

To manage your condition effectively, you must take full responsibility for your health and learn all you can about your condition.

You should quiz your doctor, go online, join online forums and local support groups, read books, and stay up-to-date with the latest news on your condition.

There's nothing wrong with regular visits to your doctor and discussing any new information or issues with them. It's to be encouraged.

The bottom line is that working with your physician you must take charge of your health and implement a plan to manage your condition.

Your journey won't be easy, especially at the start, that's for sure. And when first diagnosed you're going to go through a rollercoaster of different emotions.

Strangely enough, one of the first could be immense "relief" simply because now you know why your life has been so miserable for so long!

But then, once the reality sinks in, you can feel a sense of "grief" or even "fear" at the significant changes you'll have to make to your life, for the rest of your life. And many people will lack confidence in their ability to stay the course.

So, when first diagnosed, you need to recognize that all the different emotions you feel are normal. You are not unique and you are not alone. The key plank in your journey is to stay determined and positive throughout.

Get into a positive state of mind of knowing that going gluten-free is not a choice for you, it's an absolute necessity: the only way you are going to be well again. The hard part is over; you now know your real enemy and what to do about it. And you CAN do it; don't have any doubts about that!

Focus on how lucky you are. Yes really! You've been given the chance of a new life, free from pain and anxiety, perhaps even depression. So embrace it and accept it with open arms and, with your new positive attitude, everything else will fall into place.

But you must not forget that you have to take responsibility for your health. Your success will depend on that. So becoming very knowledgeable on your condition and everything that surrounds it is a critical part of your going gluten-free.

Below is an outline of the key steps for going gluten-free. The chapters following this one will deal with them in more detail:

Step 1

The first step is to discuss what needs to be done with your doctor who will give you valuable information on removing gluten from your life, usually accompanied by leaflets, reports, etc. They may also recommend some additional resources. You may already have done this.

Step 2

Learn all you can about your food friends and your food enemies.

Your food friends are those foods that are naturally gluten-free, e.g., fresh vegetables, fresh fruit, fresh meat and fish.

Your food enemies, clearly, are those foods that contain gluten. So you need to become an expert at reading labels on packaged, canned and pre-prepared foods and ingredients. A vital element in this is recognizing those ingredients that contain gluten but appear in the list under another name.

Step 3

This is all about making your home gluten-free. In the home there's a real danger of gluten cross-contamination from other foods, utensils, containers, work surfaces, and so on, especially when the rest of the family doesn't have a gluten problem and wishes to stay with their existing diet.

Step 4

This is an extension of step 3. You need to discuss your condition with your family and loved ones. Their understanding and support are vital to regaining your health. They need to know why gluten makes you so very ill; even the tiniest amount.

They also need to know just how dangerous cross-contamination is for you if you live together and what they'll need to do, along with you, to ensure that you don't get "glutened."

But even if you live apart, cross-contamination can be a problem when you visit their homes. How will they handle that when you are round for dinner, for example? Even stopping by for a cup of coffee or tea can be problematic.

Cross-contamination aside, you need to enlighten them about what you can and cannot eat and how to read labels to ensure that what they serve you is truly gluten-free.

Step 5

This is all about the things that need to be done to manage your condition outside of the home. For example, at work, socializing, eating out, and so on.

In the same way that you brought your family on board, you need to do the same with your work colleagues and friends, so that whether you are at work or socializing, you keep yourself safe.

Eating out can be a problem, but not as big as it once was since more and more eateries are providing gluten-free options. Once again, however, cross-contamination may be the main issue but this can be addressed by speaking to the chef or cook.

Step 6

This is where you completely redesign your daily diet to contain only gluten-free items using your knowledge gained in step 2.

This is best done by planning each meal and snack at least one week ahead, preferably a month ahead. Concentrate on using naturally gluten-free foods at first until you become an expert at recognizing non-natural gluten-free foods.

The above is a high-level look at the key issues you need to address. The chapters that follow will provide much more detail to help you transition fast and safely to your new healthy, gluten-free lifestyle.

10. IS GLUTEN-FREE THE SAME AS WHEAT-FREE?

This is a very important question with a very simple answer: NO they are NOT the same...

A product labeled "wheat-free" just means that there should be no wheat in the product, but it could still contain gluten since gluten is also found in barley and rye.

As a result, if you have gluten intolerance you shouldn't assume that wheat-free is the same as gluten-free and that food labeled "wheat-free" is safe to eat.

Likewise, someone with a wheat allergy cannot assume that a product labeled "gluten-free" would be safe, since they may be allergic to one or more of the other wheat proteins.

So, as someone with gluten intolerance, you need to look for the "gluten-free" label while somebody who is allergic to wheat needs to look for the "wheat-free" label. And where such labels do not exist you and they need to scrutinize the list of ingredients on the packaging.

11. GOING GLUTEN-FREE IN THE HOME

The key thing to bear in mind is that the tiniest bit of gluten will make you ill. So you have to be scrupulous in the home environment. Here are key steps for making and keeping a gluten-free home:

Make everyone who has access to the kitchen aware that they have a critical role in helping to keep you gluten-free.

If they wish to continue to eat gluten, cross-contamination becomes a real threat. So you'll need to keep your gluten-free stuff as far away from their stuff as possible, preferably in separate storage areas, and tightly sealed and clearly labeled.

Thoroughly clean the cupboards where the non-gluten foodstuffs are going and only use new containers with good seals for all gluten-free products.

Where non-gluten and gluten foods have to be kept refrigerated, they have to be stored separately in the fridge/freezer and labelled accordingly.

Always put gluten-free food ABOVE gluten food in refrigerators, never the other way round. The same goes for shared cupboards.

Thoroughly clean work surfaces right after every use: don't think, "I'll leave that till later."

Certain kitchenware items are hard to keep gluten-free so they will need to be bought new for the non-gluten eater and not to be shared with the gluten eater:

For example, toasters are an obvious one because they end up full of bread crumbs that are impossible to clean properly. Keep separate toasters.

Non-stick pans are another as they often end up with scratches that trap gluten, no matter how well washed. So don't share those if they've already been used, instead, the non-gluten eater should buy new ones for their own use only.

Other items that are hard to keep completely clean are colanders and sieves, where the gluten can adhere to the sides of the holes/wires and is extremely difficult to remove. New ones should be bought for the non-gluten eater.

Anything made of plastic, nylon, silicone or wood shouldn't be shared. These are things like containers, mixing bowls, chopping boards, utensils, and so on. New ones should be purchased and kept separately.

Items that don't trap gluten, and can easily be scrubbed and cleaned to eliminate all traces of gluten, may be retained. These are things like stainless steel and solid aluminum pots and pans without any non-stick coating. But they must be scrupulously cleaned right after every use. The same goes for solid metal and stainless steel utensils and cutlery.

Now, if all the other kitchen users volunteer to move to a gluten-free diet too – it happens sometimes – then it does make things much easier as cross-contamination is much less of a problem.

But you need to throw out everything that has gluten in it or has been used for gluten products. Wash everything down and start from scratch using only gluten-free products and new kitchenware items mentioned earlier.

12. GLUTEN-FREE OUTSIDE THE HOME

Many eating establishments provide excellent gluten-free options nowadays. So get to know the places in your area that do. Most of us tend to eat in just a few favorite local restaurants, so start with them.

Go in and talk to them. Ask them to show you their kitchens so you see how they handle gluten-free foods. The key thing in restaurants, cafes, bistros, etc., is the risk of cross-contamination. So talk to them about how they prevent this on their premises.

Use the same approach for your work restaurant or canteen. Let the staff know your requirements and ask how they intend to support you.

If your place of work has a small self-service kitchen that everyone uses with a microwave, fridge, toaster, coffee machine, etc., -- you know the type of thing -- then you have to treat that like your kitchen back home.

So let your colleagues know of your condition, how serious it is, and that you need their help to keep you gluten-free. Show them what needs to be done and agree on a set of rules/procedures for everyone to follow. People are very helpful, in the main.

The key thing when thinking about eating out is to plan ahead. If you're invited to a restaurant you don't know, get the telephone number and give them a ring. Talk to the chef if possible, not the manager; the chef knows his kitchen inside out.

It's the same when traveling abroad. Get a list of eateries in the area where you're going and contact them ahead of time.

13. SHOPPING FOR GLUTEN-FREE

Gluten-Free Labeling

Loose fresh fruits and vegetables, fresh meat, fresh fish, most nuts and seeds, and most dairy are naturally free from gluten. These are easy to recognize when shopping.

The problem is with processed and packaged foods. So a good understanding of labeling, and what each label means, is vital when shopping for gluten-free products.

However, until there's a universal consensus on acceptable levels of gluten, and the definitions of these levels are standardized, labeling of food and non-food products as "gluten-free" and "containing gluten ingredients" will vary from country to country.

For example, by law, in the USA, UK, Canada, and the European Union, the maximum amount of gluten allowed in a product that can be labeled "gluten-free" is 20 ppm (parts per million).

However, in Australia and New Zealand, for a product to be labeled "gluten-free," it must not contain any gluten measurable by the most sensitive test method that has universal acceptance. Some methods can measure down to 5 ppm and are improving all the time, so they really seem to be getting closer to "gluten-free."

In terms of ensuring compliance, the governing bodies in each country should carry out periodic site inspections, product testing and labeling reviews to ensure that the end product meets their specifications. They should also follow up on any customer complaints.

In addition to this, there are several independent certification bodies, such as the Gluten-Free Certification Program (GFCP) and the Gluten-Free Certification Organization (GFCO) which can provide third-party oversight and, through rigorous testing and inspection, certify that a product meets the applicable standard.

Some certification organizations apply a stricter definition of "gluten-free" than some countries' governing bodies. For example, both GFCP and GFCO define "gluten-free" as having less than 10 ppm.

Producers don't need to get certification from these bodies, but more and more are signing up because they see the benefits to their brand and their customers of having a third-party independent certification logo on their products.

This is also good for shoppers as they now have the assurance that the product they are looking at meets the gluten-free standard required by law.

It also means a much better shopping experience as they can shop without the hassle of having to ask shop assistants or, worse still, having to telephone manufacturers about their products.

Unfortunately, there isn't a universally accepted label format to identify a gluten-free product. There are hundreds of gluten-free labels out there. Even certification bodies have different labels.

There are some common factors to look out for though: many of the labels are round and one of the most popular images on them is a stalk(s) of wheat overlaid with a strike-through. They are usually accompanied by text such as "Gluten-Free" or "Certified Gluten-Free." Another favorite is to use a "tick" with the words "Gluten-Free" or "Certified Gluten-Free."

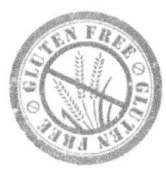 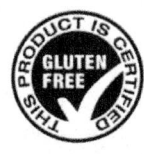 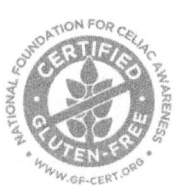

There are many different labels out there, so always double-check the ingredients listed on the package just to be sure. Note: you'll find a list of gluten-containing ingredients and additives that you might not be familiar with in the next chapter.

One final thing, there's nothing to stop unscrupulous suppliers slapping a label on their products without going through the proper certification process. One way to reduce your risk in this is to buy products from big, well-known brands, since they can't afford the bad publicity arising from mislabeling, misleading their customers and making them ill.

Foods without Gluten-Free Labeling

What about packaged foods that don't have a gluten-free label like the ones described above? How do you deal with those? Well, you just have to read the ingredients listed on the packaging.

However, even if you don't find the word "gluten" on the list that doesn't mean that it isn't in the food. It could be under a different name, in another listed ingredient, or present through cross-contamination during the manufacturing process.

At the end of the next chapter, I have listed food items that you probably wouldn't recognize as being or containing gluten, but could appear on product ingredient lists.

Do not take any risks with your health. If you aren't sure, be prepared to walk away and look for another manufacturer's product, or even in another store.

14. FOODS TO AVOID

The obvious foods to be avoided are **wheat, barley and rye.** But you must also avoid foods that contain, or usually contain, or could contain, wheat, barley or rye; it's all about risk management. For example, it's safer to avoid the following unless labeled gluten-free:

Beer	Fish in breadcrumbs	Oats (see note)
Bread	Fish in flour	Pasta
Broth	Fish in sauce	Pastries
Cakes	Flour tortillas	Salad dressings
Cereals	Fried food	Sauces
Cheese (processed, additives, beer washed)	Frozen meals	Sausages
Cookies	Gravies	Seasoned foods
Couscous	Hot dogs	Soup
Crackers	Imitation crab	Soy sauce

	meat	
Croutons	Luncheon meat	Teriyaki sauce
Dressings	Meat in breadcrumbs	Vegetables in breadcrumbs
	Meat in flour	Vegetables in flour
	Meat in sauce	Vegetables in sauce
	Muffins	

Note: Although oats don't contain gluten, they can be cross-contaminated during processing, so it may be prudent to avoid oats as well.

However, some manufacturers certify on their packaging that their oats have been milled and processed in a gluten-free environment. You may wish to keep a lookout for those in your area. Or just search online for "gluten-free oats suppliers."

Now what about foods and ingredients that you may not be familiar with? That's a real problem, isn't it? I mean, if you aren't familiar with them, how would you know whether they contained gluten or not?

Here's a list of foods and ingredients that contain gluten or have a high risk of containing gluten. So, if any of the following items appear on a list of ingredients on a product then that product should be avoided:

Artificial flavoring	Kamut	Triticale
Barley grass	Malt	Triticum spelta
Bleached flour	Malto-dextrin	Triticum vulgare
Bread flour	Modified starch	Vegetable starch
Bulgur	Natural flavoring	Wheat bran
Couscous	Seasonings	Wheat flour
Dextrin	Secale cereale	Wheat germ extract
Durum wheat	Seitan	Wheat germ oil
Farina	Semolina	Wheat grass
Flavorings	Spelt	Wheat protein

Hordeum vulgare		Wheat starch
Hydrolyzed plant protein		Whole wheat flour
Hydrolyzed vegetable protein		
Hydrolyzed wheat protein		
Hydrolyzed wheat starch		

Note: The two lists show the most common foods and ingredients to get you started. You should be able to get even more from your local support group, which I encourage you to seek out and join. There are also many forums online that have really helpful communities.

15. GLUTEN-FREE FOODS

Generally speaking, you'll be safe with fresh fruit and vegetables, fresh meat and fish, most dairy products and rice, etc., basically, anything that naturally doesn't contain gluten, hasn't been processed, and hasn't been exposed to gluten from producer to checkout.

Loose fresh fruit and vegetables are gluten-free and don't need labeling. However, be wary of pre-packed fruit and vegetables which may have been through a line that previously had gluten products on it. This is especially true for pre-cut fruit and vegetables. Stick to loose unless the packaging states that the contents are gluten-free.

Fresh meat and fish are safe but beware of pre-packed, pre-cooked, pre-coated, or pre-prepared items, unless they are labeled gluten-free.

Plain cheese should be safe as long as it's made with simple, natural ingredients and does not contain additives such as salt, flavorings, herbs, preservatives, etc., because such additives increase the risk of cross-contamination. Avoid cheese that has been "beer washed" and any other cheeses that that company makes (possible cross-contamination). Check the ingredients in every cheese to be safe.

Eggs are free of gluten, as is **milk,** but avoid flavored milk as this can contain gluten in the flavorings, unless stated otherwise. Some **milk substitutes** are safe but others are not, so check the labels very carefully.

Plain butter is gluten-free, and **plain margarine** should be too but many brands contain additives which could either contain gluten or increase the risk of cross-contamination. So, once again, read those labels!

Plain yogurt is safe, as are some flavored ones, but you need to check their labels to be on the safe side.

Beans, peas, lentils, nuts and seeds are safe to eat as long as they are plain, with no additives or coatings.

Single herbs and spices should be gluten-free. However, cross-contamination during manufacturing is a risk if the manufacturer also makes seasonings that can have additives as well as spices and herbs. So, as a safety precaution, always read the ingredients on these types of products.

There are many **gluten-free grains** that you can use as alternatives to wheat, barley and rye, but you have to eat the whole grain, i.e. with all of the bran, germ, and endosperm. Typical of these are buckwheat, millet, sorghum, quinoa, cornmeal (not corn starch!), corn, brown rice, wild rice, amaranth, teff, and

Indian rice grass (montina). And don't forget oats grown and processed in a gluten-free environment and certified gluten-free.

As more and more manufacturers and suppliers see the commercial benefits of providing gluten-free products for an ever-expanding market, more and more of our everyday foodstuffs are being made free from gluten.

So where before you had to make your own bread, cakes, cookies, snacks, sauces, soups, gravies, etc., using gluten-free substitute ingredients, nowadays you can buy many of them off the shelf. You just have to look for the certified gluten-free label.

I hope you can now appreciate just how much nutritious, healthy and delicious gluten-free food there is out there; the list is growing by the day. And as the market and competition continue to grow at a phenomenal pace, so the prices will continue to fall and bargains be had.

Finally, when shopping, if you're not sure whether a product has gluten in it or not, put it back on the shelf and move on; there are plenty more to choose from. Never take a chance with your health.

16. PRODUCTS THAT CONTAIN GLUTEN

Moving to a gluten-free lifestyle isn't just about changing your diet. Gluten can appear in the most unexpected places.

For example, many **cosmetic** and **toiletry products** contain gluten.

While it's true that -- as far as we know -- gluten is only a problem when ingested, some of these products can easily get into your digestive system via the mouth, for example, in lipstick and lip balm.

But what about gluten that can eventually be digested because of hands not being washed after touching or applying other products, such as makeup?

And there are toiletries to think about too; things like toothpaste, mouthwash, soap, shampoo, and so on.

Start with your existing products; read the ingredients to ensure they are gluten-free. If it's not obvious then contact the manufacturer. Anything that isn't should be thrown out and replaced with gluten-free alternatives.

As always when shopping, check labels and ingredients. If in doubt, ask the shop assistant, and if they don't know, ask them to contact the manufacturer. There are also many websites online that can give you the information you need.

Medications often contain gluten. These are usually in the non-active ingredients that many medications have in them. These are things like fillers which are used to give medications their shape and to help with absorption, as well as just to help bulk-up the product.

Gluten in medicines is much harder to spot. Even pharmacies can sometimes find it difficult since the ingredient might be given on the label but its name doesn't give any indication that it could be gluten-based or at risk of cross-contamination during the manufacturing process.

If you are given any medication by your doctor ask them to check their sources that it's free from gluten. Even then, double-check with the pharmacist when collecting your prescription.

Then there are **supplements**. Many of these can contain gluten in the same way as prescription or over-the-counter medications.

This is especially concerning for celiacs since they may have to use supplements to get the nutrients they've been missing. However, they should do everything in their power to get these through their new healthy gluten-free diet.

And, would you believe it, some **art supplies** contain gluten! Play-Doh and finger paints for example.

Any gluten-intolerant patient must get to know the products that contain even the minutest amount of gluten and avoid them. There are gluten-free alternatives out there: the Internet is a great place to find up-to-date information on gluten-free products and brands.

17. COPING WITH CRAVINGS

Coping with cravings can be a challenge when you transition to a gluten-free lifestyle. Whether you're tempted by the aroma of freshly baked bread or longing for your favorite pasta dish, cravings have a powerful grip. However, with the right strategies and mindset, you can manage cravings effectively while still enjoying delicious and satisfying gluten-free foods.

Understanding Cravings

Cravings are intense desires for specific foods triggered by various factors, including physiological, psychological, and environmental influences. For someone with gluten intolerance, cravings may result from withdrawal from gluten-containing foods, emotional cues, or habitual behaviors.

Recognize Triggers

The first step in managing cravings is recognizing the triggers that lead to them. These triggers can vary but may include stress, boredom, social situations, or exposure to tempting food environments. Keeping a journal to track your cravings and their associated triggers can provide valuable insights into patterns and help you develop personalized coping strategies.

Mindful Eating Practices

Practicing mindful eating can increase your awareness of hunger and satiety cues, making it easier to respond to cravings in a balanced way. Techniques such as eating slowly, savoring each bite, and paying attention to flavors and textures can help you find satisfaction in gluten-free foods. Additionally, mindfulness techniques like deep breathing, meditation, or guided imagery can help you cope with cravings as they arise.

Stock Healthy Alternatives

Keep a variety of gluten-free snacks and treats on hand to satisfy cravings without compromising your health goals. Opt for nutritious options like fresh fruit, vegetables with hummus, nuts, seeds, or Greek yogurt. Having these options readily available makes it easier for you to make healthy choices when cravings strike.

Plan Ahead

Developing a meal plan that includes balanced meals and snacks can help prevent excessive hunger and reduce the likelihood of succumbing to cravings. Batch cooking or prepping ingredients ahead of time can also make it easier for you to stick to your gluten-free diet, especially on busy days. When dining out or attending social events, research gluten-free options in advance and come prepared to make informed choices.

Develop Coping Strategies

Experiment with different distraction techniques to redirect your attention away from cravings when they arise. Engage in a hobby, go for a walk, or practice relaxation techniques to help shift your focus away from food. Find alternative ways to cope with emotions or stressors without turning to food, such as journaling, talking to a friend, or practicing mindfulness exercises.

Seek Support

Don't hesitate to reach out to friends, family, or support groups for encouragement and accountability on your gluten-free journey. Sharing experiences and coping strategies with others who understand the challenges can provide valuable support and motivation. Consulting with a registered dietitian or healthcare professional can offer personalized guidance and support tailored to your individual needs.

Celebrate Successes

Recognize and celebrate your achievements in managing cravings and sticking to your gluten-free lifestyle. Set realistic goals and milestones to track your progress and reward yourself for your hard work and dedication.

Coping with cravings on your gluten-free journey requires patience, persistence, and a willingness to try different strategies.

By understanding your triggers, practicing mindful eating, stocking healthy alternatives, and seeking support when needed, you can successfully navigate cravings while enjoying a delicious and satisfying gluten-free diet.

18. ACCIDENTAL GLUTEN INGESTION

Living with gluten intolerance requires diligence and a keen awareness of the foods you consume. However, even the most cautious can find themselves inadvertently ingesting gluten. Knowing how to manage these instances is crucial for minimizing discomfort and promoting a fast recovery.

Here are some suggestions should you find yourself glutened:

- Drink plenty of water to help flush out and rehydrate your body, especially if you have diarrhea.

- Fatigue is a common symptom after gluten ingestion, so allow your body to rest and recover.

- Ginger or peppermint herbal teas can ease and soothe upset stomachs.

- Applying heat to the abdomen can also provide relief.

- Probiotics and digestive supplements may help support gut health and alleviate symptoms.

- Over-the-counter digestive enzymes specifically formulated to aid in gluten digestion may help. But these shouldn't be relied upon as a substitute for avoiding gluten.

- Keep gluten-free snacks on hand for times when safe food options are limited.

- After being glutened, focus on consuming lighter gluten-free meals to help ease digestive discomfort and promote healing.

- If symptoms persist or worsen, consult a healthcare professional.

Accidental gluten ingestion can be frustrating, but it's important to be kind to yourself. Focus on self-care and remember that setbacks happen.

Use the incident as a learning opportunity. Reflect on what went wrong and how you can prevent similar occurrences in the future.

By taking proactive steps to manage accidental gluten ingestion, you can minimize discomfort and support your overall well-being.

Remember, prevention is key, but knowing how to respond when glutened is equally important in maintaining a healthy, gluten-free lifestyle.

19. WHAT HAVE YOU LEARNED?

If you've read right to the end then you now know more than the majority of people who have just been diagnosed with gluten intolerance.

This is important because the more knowledgeable you are about your condition, the more you can take responsibility for your health.

In this way, you'll be in a far stronger position to make that vital transition to the new you: healthy, vibrant, and full of energy.

Let's summarize what you've discovered:

The term "gluten intolerance" is used to describe a range of gluten-related conditions including celiac disease and non-celiac gluten sensitivity.

Gluten is a protein found in wheat, barley and rye, which are frequently used as ingredients in lots of food products.

Celiac disease affects about 1% of people around the world while non-celiac gluten sensitivity is thought to affect around 6%. These figures could be understated due to massive under-diagnosis.

Celiac disease is a genetic autoimmune disease where the internal lining of the small intestine gets inflamed and damaged causing malabsorption of nutrients.

There are over 300 symptoms of celiac disease, some of the most common being; weight loss, bloating, pain, diarrhea, anemia, fatigue, joint pain, osteoporosis, skin rash (dermatitis herpetiformis), anxiety, and depression.

If not properly addressed, celiac disease can lead to other serious health issues like rheumatoid arthritis, type 1 diabetes, autoimmune liver disease, lupus, non-Hodgkin lymphoma, thyroid problems, infertility and miscarriage.

Non-celiac gluten sensitivity is not an autoimmune disease so there is no damage to the small intestine although the range of symptoms is similar to celiac disease. Some experts believe that it's caused by the body's innate immune response.

Celiac disease and non-celiac gluten sensitivity should not be confused with wheat allergy which is an allergic immune response to a protein in wheat. A severe wheat allergic reaction can result in life-threatening anaphylaxis whereas celiac disease and gluten sensitivity do not.

There are recognized tests to help diagnose celiac disease (blood, endoscopy, biopsy) but not for gluten sensitivity. The only way to come to a conclusion of non-celiac gluten sensitivity is to eliminate gluten over a period, watch to see if the symptoms disappear, then gradually add gluten back into the diet and see if they re-appear.

There is no cure for celiac disease or non-celiac gluten sensitivity. The only way to manage them is through a gluten-free diet. If sufferers can stick to a gluten-free diet it has been shown that their symptoms can be alleviated and they can get their health back.

The challenge for both celiac and gluten-sensitive patients is to move to a gluten-free lifestyle both in and out of the home and stick with it.

In the home, gluten-free and gluten-containing foods must be stored in separate, well-labeled containers. To reduce cross-contamination certain appliances, tools and utensils have to be bought new and only used for gluten-free. All surfaces have to be scrupulously clean.

Eating out is easier nowadays since more and more eateries have gluten-free on their menus. It makes sense though to talk to the chefs or cooks in these places to make sure there is no risk of cross-contamination.

Shopping for gluten-free produce is also becoming much easier due to the prevalence of gluten-free produce and the introduction of gluten-free labeling.

For a manufacturer in North America, the European Union, Canada and the United Kingdom, to label a product as gluten-free, it must contain less than 20 ppm of gluten. Australia and New Zealand have even tighter regulations.

You need to study the ingredients on the packaging if you do not see a gluten-free label on a product. If in doubt ask in-store, contact the manufacturer, or contact your local support group.

There are also non-food items that may contain gluten. These are things, such as lipstick, lip balm, cosmetics, toothpaste, mouthwash, shampoo, soap, medications, supplements, and some art supplies.

To overcome food cravings as you transition, get to know your triggers, practice mindful eating, stock healthy alternatives, and seek support when needed.

Accidental glutenation is always a risk. Hydration, rest, probiotics, digestive enzymes, and lighter meals can help the body recover.

In conclusion, to regain your health you must move to a gluten-free lifestyle. It does take a lot of willpower to start with, but once you are into the swing of things, it'll become second nature.

Embrace the journey, celebrate your successes, and remember that you have the power to take control of your health and well-being.

So, starting today, take massive action, and very soon you'll be thoroughly enjoying living gluten-free!

APPENDIX A: MEAL PLANS

Here's a delicious lineup for breakfasts, lunches, dinners, and snacks to keep you fueled and satisfied throughout the day.

Start your mornings with the likes of spinach, tomato, and mushroom omelets or gluten-free pancakes.

Indulge in lunches like homemade tomato soup or grilled vegetable wraps.

For dinners, enjoy baked salmon or grilled chicken with plenty of veggies.

And don't forget to keep your energy up with nutritious snacks like fresh fruit, nuts, and rice cakes.

The key is to nourish your body with a balanced diet full of natural vitamins and minerals.

Breakfasts

- Spinach, tomato, and mushroom omelet.

- Gluten-free pancakes with maple syrup and fresh fruit.

- Natural yoghurt with raw honey and mixed berries.

- Smoked salmon with cucumber and gluten-free bagels.

- Gluten-free banana bread with natural yogurt and mixed berries.

- Frittata with spinach, cherry tomatoes, and feta cheese.

- Gluten-free cream of rice cereal with fresh fruit and nuts.

Lunches

- Stir-fried vegetables (carrots, baby sweetcorn, spring onions, cucumber, mange touts) with cashew nuts.

- Smoked haddock, grilled tomatoes and a poached egg.

- Homemade tomato soup with gluten-free bread rolls.

- Red apple and beetroot salad with salad leaves and almonds.

- Grilled vegetable and hummus wrap in a gluten-free tortilla.

- Baked potato with crabmeat, gluten-free mayo, sweetcorn, and chopped parsley.

- Bean and cheese burritos made with corn tortillas.

Dinners

- Baked salmon with steamed broccoli and quinoa.

- Roasted red pepper risotto with natural brown risotto rice, vegetable stock, wine.

- Grilled chicken breast with boiled potatoes, carrots and parsnips.

- Homemade Irish stew.

- Grilled steak with roasted potatoes and green beans.

- Baked or grilled hake with salsa verde and steamed vegetables.

- Grilled pork chops, sweet potato mash and roasted Brussels sprouts.

Snacks

3 snacks a day: one mid-morning, one mid-afternoon and one in the evening.

- 1 cup of fresh cherries.
- 1 cup of fresh berries.
- 1/3 cup of dried apricots.

- 1/3 cup of almonds.

- 1/3 cup whole sesame seeds.

- 1/3 cup of pecan nuts.

- 1/3 cup of mixed dried fruit and nuts.

- 1/3 cup of mixed nuts.

- Plain rice cakes with peanut butter.

- Rice crackers with guacamole.

- Celery sticks with cream cheese.

- Carrot sticks with hummus.

- Plain popcorn with oil and salt.

- Gluten-free pretzels with dipping mustard.

These are only suggestions. The important thing is to eat a balanced diet with plenty natural vitamins and minerals to help your body heal itself and stay healthy.

APPENDIX B: POSITIVE AFFIRMATIONS

Living with gluten intolerance might throw some curveballs your way, but it's also a chance to discover new paths to wellness and happiness. These affirmations are like little pep talks, reminding you of your strength, positivity, and dedication to taking care of yourself.

Whether you're navigating social situations, trying out tasty gluten-free recipes, or just listening to your body, these affirmations are here to cheer you on and help you embrace your gluten-free journey with a smile on your face and confidence in your heart. You've got this!

"I embrace my gluten intolerance as a pathway to better health and vitality."

"I choose foods that nourish and support my body, free from gluten."

"My gluten intolerance does not define me; it empowers me to make healthier choices."

"I am grateful for the opportunity to explore new, delicious gluten-free recipes and foods."

"I trust my body's wisdom and respect its needs, including avoiding gluten."

"Living gluten-free allows me to prioritize my well-being and live my best life."

"I am resilient and adaptable, finding joy and satisfaction in my gluten-free lifestyle."

"Every day, I discover more ways to enjoy life fully while honoring my gluten intolerance."

"I am in control of my health and happiness, making informed choices that support my gluten-free journey."

"My gluten intolerance challenges me to be creative, resourceful, and open-minded, leading to a richer and more fulfilling life."

"I am grateful for the growing awareness and availability of gluten-free options, making my journey easier."

"My body thrives on wholesome, nourishing gluten-free foods, promoting my overall well-being."

"I honor my body's signals and prioritize self-care by steering clear of gluten-containing products."

"Every day, I celebrate my gluten-free lifestyle as a journey toward optimal health and vitality."

"I release any attachment to gluten and embrace the abundance of delicious, gluten-free alternatives."

"My gluten intolerance inspires me to prioritize mindful eating and cultivate a deeper connection with my body."

"I radiate positivity and resilience, effortlessly navigating social situations while staying true to my gluten-free needs."

"I am supported by a community of fellow gluten-free individuals, sharing experiences, recipes, and encouragement."

"My gluten intolerance is a blessing in disguise, guiding me toward a more conscious and fulfilling way of living."

"I am proud of my commitment to my health and well-being, thriving and flourishing on my gluten-free journey."

APPENDIX C: RESOURCES

These resources aim to educate and assist those affected by gluten-related disorders:

- https://www.niddk.nih.gov/health-information/digestive-diseases/celiac-disease

- https://www.webmd.com/digestive-disorders/celiac-disease/features/gluten-intolerance-against-grain

- https://www.nhs.uk/conditions/coeliac-disease/

- https://www.massgeneral.org/children/celiac-disease/gluten-sensitivity-faq

- https://www.mayoclinic.org/diseases-conditions/celiac-disease/symptoms-causes/syc-20352220

- https://www.hopkinsmedicine.org/health/conditions-and-diseases/celiac-disease

- https://www.celiac.ca/

- https://coeliac.org.au/learn/coeliac-disease/

- https://coeliac.org.nz/

- https://www.beyondceliac.org/celiac-disease/non-celiac-gluten-sensitivity/

- https://www.coeliac.org.uk/information-and-support/coeliac-disease/about-coeliac-disease/gluten-sensitivity/

- https://celiac.org/

Printed in Dunstable, United Kingdom